Seydou Amadou TRAORE

BCG, VAR1, Penta3 vaccination coverage in children aged 0-23 months

Seydou Amadou TRAORE

BCG, VAR1, Penta3 vaccination coverage in children aged 0-23 months

Determinants of routine vaccination

Imprint

Any brand names and product names mentioned in this book are subject to trademark, brand or patent protection and are trademarks or registered trademarks of their respective holders. The use of brand names, product names, common names, trade names, product descriptions etc. even without a particular marking in this work is in no way to be construed to mean that such names may be regarded as unrestricted in respect of trademark and brand protection legislation and could thus be used by anyone.

Cover image: www.ingimage.com

This book is a translation from the original published under ISBN 978-620-6-70671-7.

Publisher:
Sciencia Scripts
is a trademark of
Dodo Books Indian Ocean Ltd. and OmniScriptum S.R.L publishing group

120 High Road, East Finchley, London, N2 9ED, United Kingdom
Str. Armeneasca 28/1, office 1, Chisinau MD-2012, Republic of Moldova, Europe
Printed at: see last page
ISBN: 978-620-7-76344-3

Signing sessions

I dedicate this work to :

My late father: I wish you could have been there to see the results of the education and values you gave us. Rest in peace, Dad.

My mothers: thank you for all the love you give me;

My brothers and sisters: your unconditional support has made this work possible;

My wife: may this job help us to continue our wonderful family life;

Thanks

First of all, I give thanks to Allah, the All-Merciful, the Most Merciful, who is at the beginning and the end of all things, for all the blessings without which no one could exist. I pray on His beloved, the seal of the prophets, the best of creatures Mohammad (pbuh), on his family, his noble companions and all those who will follow him until the end of time.

I would like to express my sincere thanks :

To our supervisor: Pr Hamadoun SANGHO, Professor of Public Health, Preventive Medicine, Head of the Department of Teaching and Research in Public Health. You have agreed to supervise this work despite your many duties. We are sincerely grateful to you for everything you have done for us, and we would like to express our deepest gratitude.

To our co-supervisor: Dr Cheick Abou COULIBALY, MD, MPH,

Épidémiologie, Maitre-assistant en Epidémiologie au Département d'Enseignement et de Recherche en Santé Publique. Thank you for agreeing to accompany us throughout this work. Your determination and invaluable advice have enabled us to deepen our knowledge. Please accept the expression of our deepest gratitude.

To the members of the Jury :

Pr Ousmane TOURE, Director of Environmental Health Research.

Dear Maitre, You have accepted to be President of the Jury of this work in spite of your multiple tasks, we address you our sincere gratitude for everything and receive here the expression of our deep gratitude.

Dr Birama Apho LY, Senior Lecturer in Public and Community Health, Director of the Centre d'analyse Sahélo-saharienne at the Ecole de Maintien de la Paix.

Dear Maitre, You have agreed to be a member of the Jury for this work, despite your many duties. We are sincerely grateful to you for everything you have done, and we would like to express our deepest gratitude.

To all the faculty of the Department of Teaching and Research in Public Health: For their generosity and great patience despite their academic and professional responsibilities. Thank you for your teaching.

To the Mopti Health District team: Dr Issa DIARRA, Gynecologist/Obstetrician and District Chief Medical Officer, thank you for your frank collaboration.

The SIS/PEV/SE Support Doctor, the EPI/Surveillance and SIS Officers, thank you for your support and thank you again.

To Class 10: I'd like to extend my warmest thanks to the students of the Master in Public Health Class 10M2 for their courage, team spirit and generosity during the two years of training.

To all those who, from far and near, have constantly supported me during my years of study, particularly my family in general, and a special mention to my dear wife for her encouragement, patience, moral support and prayers on my behalf; please find here, through this modest work, the expression of my deepest gratitude.

Summary

Introduction : The Mopti Health District is aware of some of the factors influencing its vaccination coverage, which are rarely measured in the population as a whole. [1]. When they are significant, many children miss out on vaccination, leading to complications. The aim of the study was to investigate the factors influencing low BCG, VAR1 and Penta3 vaccination coverage among children aged 0 to 23 months in the Mopti health district in 2021.

Methodology: We carried out a descriptive cross-sectional study, collecting information on 280 selected mothers, who were questioned about immunization service provision, vaccines received by the child before the age of two and reasons for incompleteness using a questionnaire. Multivariate backward logistic regression analysis was performed for variables when p < 0.2 at univariate analysis using SPSS software. An association was significant when p < 0.05.

Results: Vaccination completeness was 53.08%, ranging from 94% for BCG to 79% for VAR1, 26% for VAR2, 103% for Penta1 and 83% for Penta3. The analysis showed that mothers who spent more time at the vaccination center (P=0.686), who missed certain vaccination sessions (P=0.357) and who were informed of shortages of consumables (P=0.161) were significantly associated with vaccine incompleteness.

Conclusion: Vaccination completeness was inadequate, despite mothers' good knowledge of vaccination.

Key words: Vaccination coverage, associated factors, EPI, district, Mali

List of acronyms / Abbreviations

WHO: World Health Organization

UNICEF: United Nations Children's Fund

EPI: Expanded Programme on Immunization

DGSHP-SI: Direction Générale de la Santé et de l'Hygiène Publique-Section d'Immunisation (Health and Public Hygiene Department - Immunization Section)

DRS: Direction Régionale de la Santé (Regional Health Department)

CSREF: Centre de Santé de Référence

USTTB: University of Technical Sciences and Technologies of Bamako

FMOS: Faculty of Medicine and Stomatology

BCG: Bacille Calminte et Guérin vaccine

VAR1: Measles vaccine 1ère dose

VAR2: Measles vaccine second dose

Penta: Pentavalent vaccine (Diphtheria, Pertussis, Hepatitis, Hemophilus and Tetanus)

VAA: Vaccin anti amaril

PCV13: Pneumococcal 13 vaccine

IPV1: Inactive polio vaccine 1ère dose

IPV2: Inactive polio vaccine second dose

Rotateq/Rotasiil: Rotavirus vaccine

IM: Intramuscular

MAPI: Manifestation Adverse Post Immunisation

DTC: Centre Technical Manager

ASACO: Community Health Association

CAFO: Coordination of Women's Associations and NGOs

Table of contents

1   Introduction :

Immunization is recognized as one of the most effective measures for preventing mortality, morbidity and complications of infectious diseases in children. [1]. Immunization coverage indicates the proportion of the target population having received the required doses of a vaccine against a preventable disease [2]. It is an important indicator of population health, and reflects the degree of susceptibility to vaccine-preventable diseases [[3,4]. It can also be used as a proxy to study the factors influencing accessibility to health services and vaccination-related interventions, providing a rapid study of the improvement or deterioration of health services [[5]. Vaccination coverage levels are required to achieve the goals of reducing vaccine-preventable diseases, and it is essential to continuously monitor the various measures of vaccine coverage [6].

Factors influencing vaccination coverage are rarely measured in the general population, but rather in specific groups in which vaccination is recommended. [7]. When they are high, many children miss out on vaccination, leading to complications from infectious diseases. It is estimated that around 3 million deaths are prevented each year worldwide thanks to vaccination, and that in addition, every year, it prevents almost 750,000 children from suffering serious physical, mental or neurological handicaps [7,8] .

In May 1974, the World Health Organization (WHO) launched a global immunization program, known as the Expanded Program on Immunization (EPI), as one of the major public health interventions to prevent childhood morbidity and mortality. The EPI aims to immunize children worldwide to prevent disease, reduce disability and death from vaccine-preventable diseases [2,9].

The Global Strategy Vision 2006 - 2015 and Program for Immunization to 2030, developed by WHO and UNICEF and adopted by the 56th session of the WHO Regional Committee for Africa, envisions a world in which every child, adolescent and adult has equitable access to immunization services. It also recommends achieving a national immunization coverage rate of at least 95%. [10-12].

In Africa, studies have shown that immunization status, the child's place of birth and residence, birth rank, the number of children in the family and the mother's education are determinants of immunization status in children. [13-18].

Failure to take these determinants of immunization status into account in the design of vaccination strategies and policies could annihilate the efforts made to achieve immunization coverage targets, and despite the mobilization of numerous human, financial and material resources, vaccine-preventable diseases would continue to claim victims. [19].

In Mali, since 2012, many factors have influenced immunization coverage, despite the implementation of the Expanded Program on Immunization (EPI), which sets an immunization coverage target for all routine antigens, including Vitamin A, of at least 95% at national level according to the immunization schedule [1,20,21].

The Mopti health district is the largest of the eight districts in the Mopti region, and according to district data, vaccination coverage was :

- 2018: 100.41% BCG vs 89.97% VAR1, 109.48% Penta1 vs 91.19% Penta3 [22];

- 2019: 98.39% BCG vs. 85.32% VAR1, 104.22% Penta1 vs. 83.16% Penta3 [22] ;

- **2020:** 94.55% BCG versus 77.78% VAR1 and 25.89% VAR2, 103.49% Penta1 versus 80.43% Penta3 [22].

In this year 2021, the district has experienced measles epidemics with 69 suspected cases for 35 positive cases, 2 suspected cases of yellow fever and 11 cases of acute flaccid paralysis; the first outbreak of cases took place from April to June with 0 deaths [22].

Despite these epidemics and this vaccination coverage, to our knowledge no study has been carried out in the Mopti health district to determine the factors influencing vaccination coverage using a standardized method, or the reasons why children are not vaccinated.

2   Lalonde's conceptual framework:

We used this framework model according to Lalonde as an analytical tool to explain the relationships between dependent and independent variables in order to obtain an overall understanding of the factors influencing low BCG, VAR1 and Penta3 vaccination coverage in the Mopti Health District in 2021 [23].

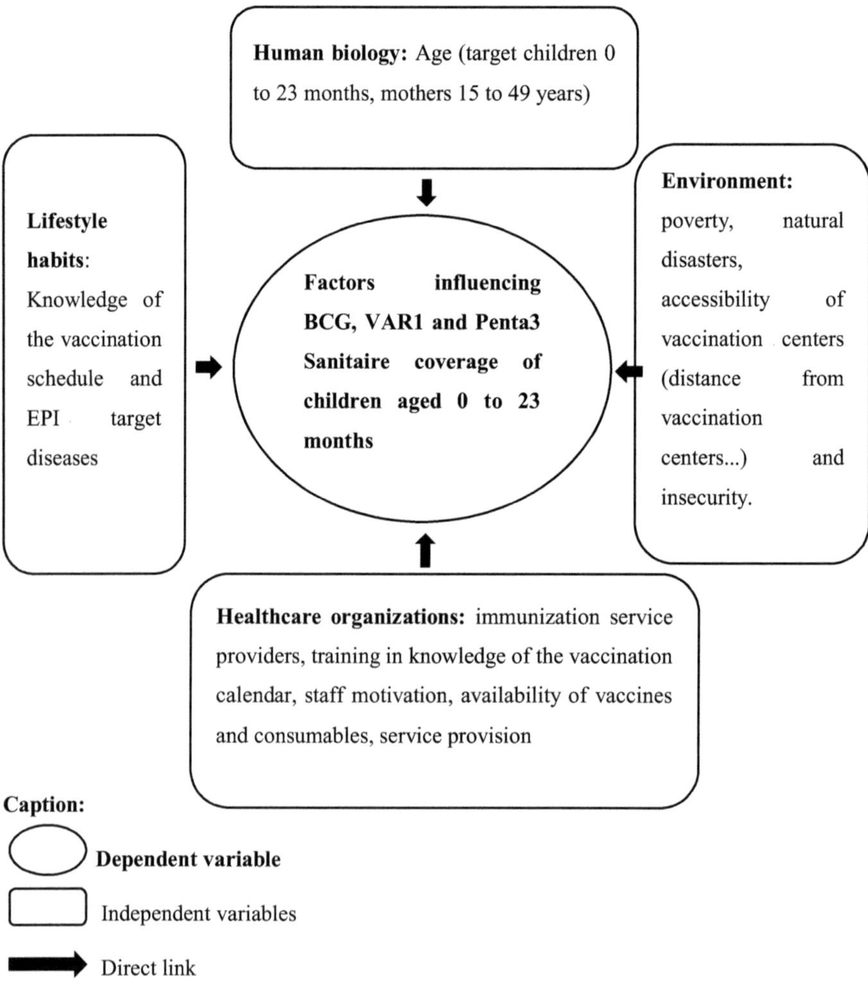

Figure 1: Conceptual framework of factors influencing immunization coverage of children aged 0 to 23 months

Explanation of the conceptual framework of factors influencing vaccination coverage :

Lifestyle habits include knowledge of the vaccination schedule and EPI target diseases. [24].

Human biology Age (children aged 0 to 23 months, babysitters or mothers of children aged 0 to 23 months and aged 15 to 49) [21].

The environment is made up of poverty, natural disasters, the accessibility of vaccination centers and insecurity. [25].

Healthcare organizations are made up of immunization service providers, training, motivation of immunization personnel, availability of vaccines and consumables, immunization service provision, etc. [26].

Based on a review of the literature, we note that knowledge, reasons for non-vaccination, accessibility of vaccination centers, poverty, health services and the provision of vaccination services by health workers are factors that can directly influence vaccination coverage of children aged 0 to 23 months [11,20,27].

We carried out literature reviews to analyze and critically evaluate a range of works. These helped to demonstrate the validity of our project, but also to clearly formulate our research question.

3.1   EPI documents from the immunization section

3.1.1   Historical reminder of the EPI :

The Expanded Program on Immunization is managed by the Immunization Section, a sub-department of the Directorate General of Health and Public Hygiene (DGSHP-SI).

It has undergone a great deal of evolution from its inception to the present day, in three main phases:

a. Phase 1 "the sweep": from 1986 to 1991

- Targets were children aged 0 to 6 and pregnant women;

- The strategies applied were both fixed and mobile;

b. Phase 2 "maintenance": 1992 to 1996

- Targets were children aged 0 to 23 months, pregnant women and women of childbearing age;

- Strategies were fixed, advanced and mobile;

c. Phase 3 "Consolidation": since 1997

- Targets were children aged 0-11 months, pregnant women and women of childbearing age;

- Strategies were fixed, advanced and mobile

New vaccines will be introduced between 2001 and 2021

- 2001: the advent of the yellow fever vaccine /VAA

- 2003: Hepatitis B vaccine introduced

- Between 2005 and 2007: Haemophilus influenzae type B (Hib)/Pentavalent vaccine (DTP-HepB-Hib) is introduced

The introduction and some reinforcement of certain antigens are definitely carried out from the capital to the rest of the country:

- In 2005: It was for the capital Bamako
- In 2006: It was the regional capitals
- In 2007: It was for the rest of the country
- 2011: Pneumococcal vaccine (PCV-13) is introduced

Between 2014 and 2015: The rotavirus diarrhea vaccine was introduced in two phases:

- In 2014: It was for the capital Bamako,
- In 2015: It was for the rest of the country
- 2016: Introduction of inactivated polio vaccine (IPV)
- In 2017: The introduction of the meningococcal A vaccine
- In 2019: It was the introduction of the second dose of VAR
- 2021: Introduction of the second dose of IPV

3.1.2 EPI target diseases in Mali :

We present some target diseases and their prevention with vaccines for the 0 to 23 months age group in Mali.

Target diseases	Vaccines
Tuberculosis	BCG
Poliomyelitis	VPO, VPI
Diphtheria, Tetanus, Pertussis, Hemophilus influenza type b, Hepatitis B	Penta (combined DTP-Hib-HepB vaccine)
Pneumonia	PCV-13
Rotavirus diarrhea	Rotateq/Rotasiil
Meningococcal meningitis A	MenA
Yellow fever	VAA
Measles	VAR

3.1.3 Immunization schedule for children aged 0 to 23 months in Mali :

Mali's updated vaccination schedule for children aged 0 to 23 months calls for the reinforcement or extension of immunity conferred by various vaccines, as well as one or more booster doses. Over time, the level of antibodies present in the body decreases. Adherence to the vaccination schedule is very important, and also means that a booster shot is necessary when mothers miss an appointment. Simply repeat the schedule and complete the injections. The duration of protection conferred by a vaccine varies. In the case of vaccines (Penta, Pneumo, Rota and Polio), the primary vaccination consists of three injections spaced one month apart over the course of the trimester. [28,29].

AGE	ANTIGENES	INJECTION ROUTES	ADMINISTRATION SITES
Birth	BCG + OPV 0	BCG = intradermal Polio = oral	Left forearm
6 weeks	Penta1+VPO1+ Pneumo1+ Rota1	Penta = IM Pneumo : IM VPO, Rota = oral	1/3 medium anterolateral thigh mouth
10 weeks	Penta2+VPO2+ Pneumo2+ Rota2	Penta = IM Pneumo : IM VPO, Rota = oral	1/3 medium anterolateral thigh mouth
14 weeks	Penta3+VPO3+ Pneumo3+ Rota3+ VPI 1	Penta = IM Pneumo : IM VPI : IM VPO, Rota = oral	1/3 medium anterolateral thigh mouth
9 to 11 months	VAR1+VAA+MenA+VPI2	Subcutaneous/IM	Upper arm (deltoid)
15 to 23 months	VAR2	Subcutaneous/IM	Upper arm (deltoid)

3.2   Study of vaccine coverage and associated factors

Vaccination is still the best way to fight the most deadly childhood diseases, especially in developing countries. [7]. In Mali, low vaccination coverage contributes to the persistence of these diseases in the country. Our study focused on identifying the factors influencing low vaccination coverage in the Mopti Health District:

According to Ba Pouth et al. Following two measles epidemics with a vaccine completeness rate of 69% according to district data. A study was conducted to determine vaccine coverage and factors associated with vaccine non-completeness in children aged 12 to 23 months in the Djoungolo-Cameroon health district in 2012. The results showed that vaccine completeness was 64.3%, ranging from 85.7% for BCG to 66.2% for measles vaccine. In conclusion, the district's vaccination coverage fell short of targets, leading the investigator to make a recommendation to strengthen parent education and reorganize vaccination services. [20].

According to Francis et al. An assessment of vaccination coverage and factors associated with vaccination status were carried out in 2017 among children in rural areas of Vellore South India. Results showed that 643 children included, vaccination coverage of children with vaccination cards (n = 606) i.e. 70.8% of children had received all doses recommended according to the UIP calendar. In conclusion, there was higher UIP antigenic coverage and a higher proportion of fully vaccinated children than previously reported in rural Vellore. [27].

According to Sangaré et al. A household survey in the health district of Ségou, Mali, 2019 to determine concordance of vaccination status and factors associated with incomplete vaccination showed that 18.46% of children were incompletely vaccinated. Mothers correctly reported their children's vaccination status in 67.30% of cases. The results showed good concordance of vaccination status. Living in a rural area, lack of education, lack of knowledge of EPI target diseases, lack of knowledge of the vaccination schedule and lack of knowledge of the importance of vaccination were factors associated with incomplete vaccination of children. [11].

4   Research question:

What factors will influence vaccination coverage among children aged 0 to 23 months in the Mopti health district in 2021?

5   Research hypothesis:

Mothers' waiting time at the center for vaccination, mothers' long waiting times for vaccination and mothers' failure to attend vaccination sessions are factors influencing BCG, VAR1 and Penta3 vaccination coverage in children aged 0 to 23 months.

6   Objectives :

6.1   General objective:

To study the factors influencing low vaccination coverage among children aged 0 to 23 months in the Mopti health district in 2021.

6.2   Specific objectives:

- Describe the District's immunization healthcare organization;
- Determine mothers' perceptions of the vaccination schedule and EPI target diseases;
- Determine the immunization coverage rate of children aged 0 to 23 months in the District;
- Identify potential factors influencing vaccination in the Mopti health district in 2021.

7 Methodologies :

7.1 Study framework:

The Mopti Health District is bordered to the north by the Niafunké District, to the northeast by the Douentza District, to the northwest by the Youwarou District, to the west by the Ténenkou District, to the east by the Bandiagara District and to the south by the Djénné District.

This study was carried out in households in the Mopti health district, one of eight health districts in the Mopti region, comprising thirty health areas of difficult accessibility, three of which are non-functional. It covers an area of 40 km^2 for a health population estimated at 535,224 in 2021, with a vaccinated population of 21,409 children aged 0-11 months and 12-23 months, and 256,908 under-15s.

Mapping the Mopti District :

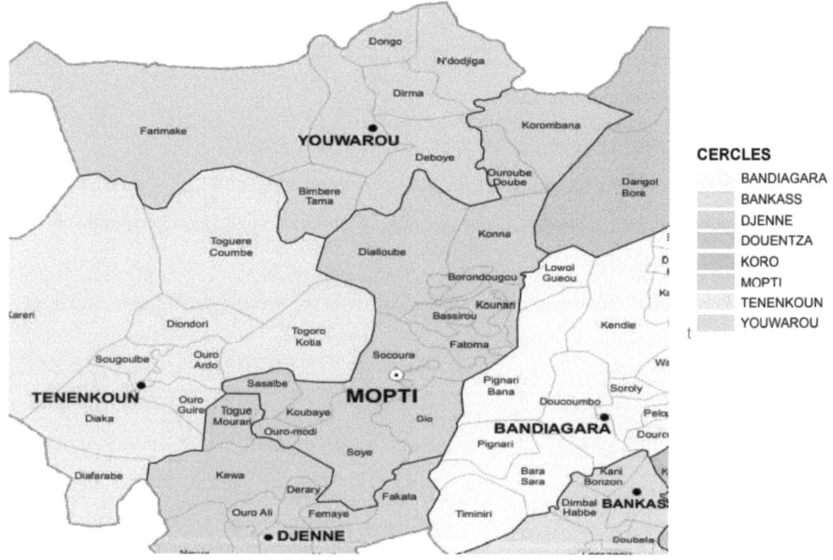

Caption:

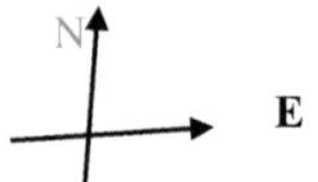

7.2 Type and period of study:

We carried out a descriptive cross-sectional study by cluster sample household survey and interview of health staff and mothers of children 0 to 23 months seen in vaccination for convenience. Data collection was carried out from November 25, 2021 to September 30, 2022.

7.3 Study population:

For the household survey, women with a child under 24 months were selected for the cluster survey.

The staff interview concerned health workers involved in vaccination activities, and part of the interview also concerned mothers of children seen in vaccination for convenience in the surveyed facilities at the time of the interview and vaccination observations.

7.4 Study design:

The study was conducted in three phases. During the first phase, a presentation of the protocol was made to the Mopti Regional Health Director and his staff, as well as to all the Chief Medical Officers of the Region's eight health districts. A meeting bringing together health authorities, DTCs, ASACO presidents, community leaders, CAFO and the press was also held in the Mopti District to obtain community approval. The second phase consisted in identifying the target group to be surveyed. The third phase is marked by the study of the influencing factors themselves.

7.4.1 Inclusion criteria:

The study included:

- Mothers of children of childbearing age (15 - 49) and with a child under 24 months in the Health District;

- Health workers involved in vaccination activities.

7.4.2 Non-inclusion criteria:

Excluded from the study :

- Mothers of children on site or with a last child over 24 months old;

- Refusal to consent to the study (mothers of children under 24 months, health workers).

7.5 Sampling:

7.5.1 Sampling procedure:

A sampling method is used:

- The probabilistic method was used to select mothers of volunteer children attending the vaccination service for convenience,

- The reasoned non-probabilistic method for observations of vaccination sessions and convenience for vaccination officers,

- The cluster survey was carried out for the household survey.

7.5.2   Sample size:

The sample size is 380 mothers of children aged 0 to 23 months with a margin of error of 10% of a 95% confidence interval for a risk α= 5%, a prevalence of 45% and calculated from Epi info version 7.2.1.0. (30) or Daniel SCHWART's formula: **n = z² x p (1 - p) / m² n = sample size z** = confidence **level**
We surveyed 5 vaccinators and observed 5 vaccination sessions.

7.6   Data collection technique

Mothers of children aged 0 to 23 months attending the vaccination service, vaccinators and observation of vaccination sessions were interviewed.

7.7   Data collection tools:

Two questionnaires have been developed:

- A questionnaire was sent to mothers of children aged 0 to 23 months. The questionnaire covered the mothers' profile, the children's vaccination status, the mothers' knowledge and perception of vaccination, and the various reasons for non-vaccination;

- A questionnaire was sent to vaccination service providers on the organization of vaccination services.

The study began with a two-day pre-survey to assess the feasibility of the survey, check acceptability and improve data collection tools. A supervisor was identified. The supervisor and the interviewers were trained in questionnaire administration for one day.

Defining variables :

The dependent variable was factors influencing low antigen-specific vaccination coverage (BCG, VAR1 and Penta3) of children aged 0 to 23 months. A child was considered fully vaccinated if he or she had received all 06 doses of the following vaccines before the age of 24 months: BCG, Penta1, Penta2, Penta3, VAR1, VAA and VAR2, according to the vaccination card and/or mother's declarations. Vaccination coverage by antigen was defined as the ratio of the number of children aged 0 to 23 months who received this antigen before the age of 24 months to the total number of children aged 0 to 23 months surveyed.

The independent variables were human biology, lifestyle, healthcare organization, environment and mothers' knowledge, attitudes and practices towards vaccination.

7.8 Data analysis technique:

All survey data were collected on tablets using the Kobocollect mobile application and uploaded daily to the Direction Nationale de la Santé et de l'Hygiène Publique for processing and validation. They were then imported into SPSS version 25 software (SPSS Inc., Chicago, IL). Data are expressed as frequency for qualitative data, and as median or mean and standard deviation for quantitative data. The association between vaccination and predictors (independent variables) was measured using logistic regression in univariate and multivariate analysis. A statistical significance level of 5% is considered for the univariate analysis, and also as an entry criterion for the multivariate stepwise model. Odds ratios and 95% confidence intervals (CI) are used to measure the risk of non-use of vaccination, and an association is significant when $p < 0.05$.

7.9 Ethical considerations:

The study protocol was submitted to the Ethics Committee of the USTTB Faculty of Medicine and Odontostomatology for approval prior to implementation.

Consent form: Those wishing to participate in the study, as well as parents or guardians of children under 24 months of age, are invited to sign the consent form.

Study staff read the information sheet and consent form, and gave all necessary explanations on these sheets, with a view to a better understanding of the study's aims and procedures. It was explained to the trained study staff that participation is voluntary and can be withdrawn at any time during the study, and that access to health care is not dependent on participation in the study. Only participants who sign the written informed consent form are enrolled.

Left index fingerprints are considered a legal document of consent in Mali, and are therefore accepted in place of a signature for illiterate people.

Anyone asked to participate in in-depth interviews with key informants or in focus groups provided verbal consent.

Confidentiality: No study participant has been identified by name in any report or publication resulting from the information collected for the study. All personal identifiers are removed from the data when it is entered. Data collection forms are kept in a storage area that complies with good clinical practice.

Risks to participants: There were no major risks to participants in enrolling (or not enrolling) in this study. Enrolled babysitters spent about 10 extra minutes answering the questionnaire.

We collected information on 280 mothers or carers of children aged 0 to 23 months to study the factors influencing low vaccination coverage, using mixed sampling. The frequencies of fully vaccinated children were 26.4% (74/280), incompletely vaccinated children 69.3% (194/280) and never vaccinated children 4.3% (12/280).

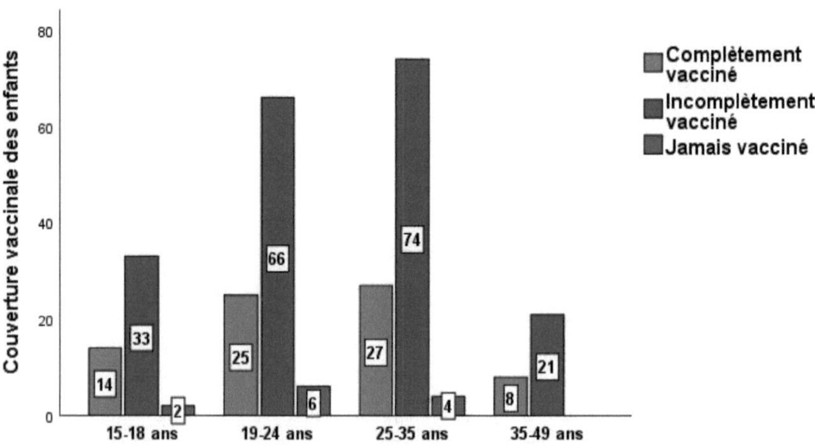

Figure 2: Vaccination coverage rate for children aged 0 to 23 months, by mother's age group

Coverage varies according to the questioning of mothers or babysitters and the availability of vaccination cards. Mothers aged 25-35 had the highest number of incompletely vaccinated children (74), compared with (27) fully vaccinated children.

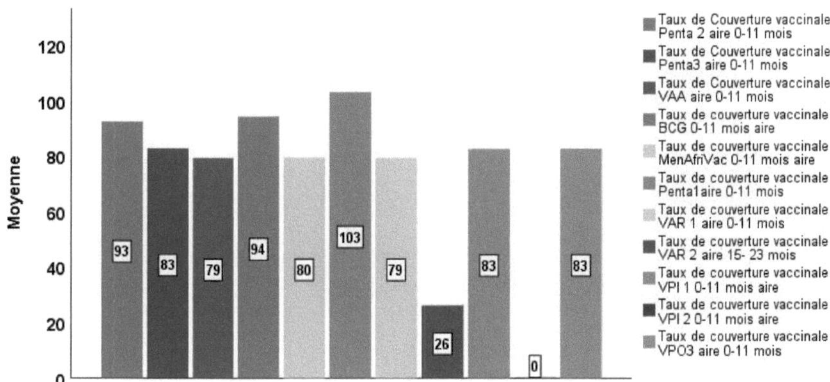

Figure 3: Rate of antigen-specific vaccination coverage of children aged 0 to 23 months in Mopti District in 2021, based on survey results and data

Antigen-specific vaccine coverage according to vaccination card and mother/caregiver declarations was : 94% (BCG), 103% (Penta1), 93% (Penta2), 83% (Penta3), 79% (VAR1), 26% (VAR2) and 79% (VAA).

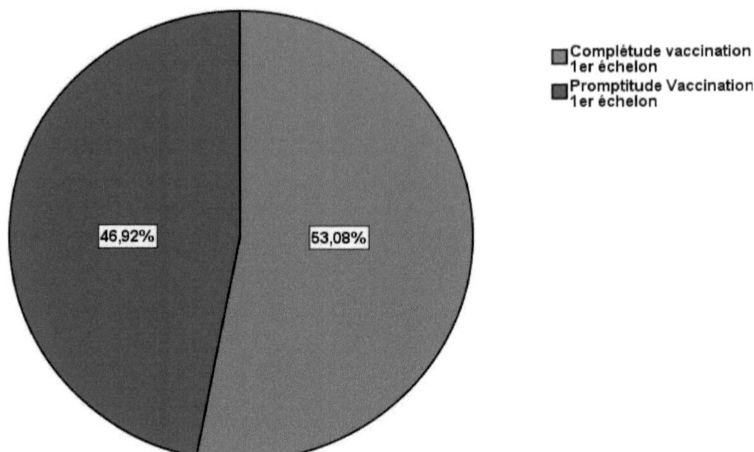

Figure 4: Vaccine completeness/accuracy in Mopti District in 2021

In 2021, District completeness/completeness falls short of the desired 100% target.

Table 1: Socio-demographic characteristics of mothers or babysitters

Variables		Number of employees (N)	Marginal percentage
Age of mother or babysitter	15-18 years	49	17,5
	19-24 years old	97	34,6
	25-35 years	105	37,5
	35-49 years	29	10,4
Mother's or babysitter's level of education	No	51	18,2
	Primary	121	43,2
	Secondary	97	34,6
	Superior	11	3,9
Mother's or janitor's occupation	Artisane	5	1,8
	Other	7	2,5
	Retailer	75	26,8
	Grower	3	1,1
	Student	18	6,4
	Student	3	1,1
	Housekeeper	169	60,4
Marital status	Single	5	1,8
	Bride	67	23,9
	Lives with a partner	208	74,3

The age groups of mothers 25 to 35 years 105(37.5%) and 19 to 24 years 97(34.6%) were the most represented, of which 121(43.2%) were in primary school and 97(34.6%) in secondary school; the household profession 169(60.4%) was dominant, of which 208(74.3%) lived as a couple.

Table 2: Socio-demographic characteristics of children aged 0 to 23 months

Variables		Number of employees (N)	Marginal percentage
Child age groups	0 - 11 months	171	61,1
	12 - 23 months	109	38,9
Children's status	Female	142	50,7
	Male	138	49,3
Child's vaccination status	Fully vaccinated	74	26,4
	Incompletely vaccinated	194	69,3
	Never vaccinated	12	4,3

The 0-11 months age group was the most represented, with 171 (61.1%) compared with 109 (38.92%) in the 12-23 months age group, 142 (50.7%) of whom were female and 138 (49.3%) male.

Table 3: Vaccination status of children by mother's level of education

Variables		Child's vaccination status		
		Fully vaccinated	Incompletely vaccinated	Never vaccinated
Mother's or babysitter's level of education	No	6	38	7
	Primary	36	82	3
	Secondary	27	68	2
	Superior	5	6	0
Total		74	194	12

Pearson Chi² = 19.946[a] , p = 0.003. Most of our children, including (82) incompletely vaccinated children and (36) fully vaccinated children, were born to mothers with primary education, compared with (7) never vaccinated children born to mothers with no schooling.

Table 4: Mothers' or babysitters' assessment of vaccination

Variables		Number of employees (N)	Marginal percentage
Age groups of mothers or babysitters	15-18 years	49	17,5
	19-24 years old	97	34,6
	25-35 years	105	37,5
	35-49 years	29	10,4
Mothers' knowledge of child immunization	Against disease	273	97,5
	Don't know	7	2,5
The benefits of vaccination	Vaccination is free	22	7,8
	Vaccination is a good thing	82	29,3
	Vaccination protects children	176	62,9
Vaccination information sources	Health center	140	52,0
	Mosque/Church	69	24,6
	Markets/neighbours	71	23,4

Most mothers, 280 (97.5%), knew why children should be vaccinated and about the Expanded Programme on Immunization (EPI), only 7 (2.5%) were unaware of it, and 62.9% knew of its benefits. The Mosque/Church was the main source of information (24.6%) in rural areas, against 52.0% from the Health Centre, followed by Markets/neighbours (23.4%) with a 95% Confidence Interval (CI) for a risk α of 0.05.

Table 5: Completion rates for children aged 0 to 23 months in Mopti District

Variables		Number of employees (N)	Marginal percentage
Child's vaccination status	Fully vaccinated	74	26,4
	Incompletely vaccinated	194	69,3
	Never vaccinated	12	4,3
Vaccination Card Availability	No	12	4,3
	Yes	268	95,7
Vaccinated child (at least one dose)	No	12	4,3
	Yes	268	95,7
According to Card	No	12	4,3
	Yes	268	95,7
According to card + mother/caregiver declarations	No	12	4,3
	Yes	268	95,7

According to the vaccination card and mother/guardian declarations, 74 (26.4%) were fully vaccinated, 194 (69.3%) were partially vaccinated and 12 (4.3%) had received no vaccine at all.

Table 6: Vaccination coverage by vaccination status

Variables		Number of employees (N)	Marginal percentage
Vaccination coverage	Fully vaccinated	74	26,4
	Incompletely vaccinated	194	69,3
	Never vaccinated	12	4,3

The majority of children, 194 (69.3%), were incompletely vaccinated, compared with 12 (4.3%) who had never been vaccinated. 95% CI for a risk α of 0.05.

Table 7: Factors associated with incomplete vaccination in relation to age

Variables		Number of employees (N)	Marginal percentage
Waiting time at the vaccination center	1-2h	28	10,0
	2-3h	192	68,6
	3-4h	49	17,5
	minus 1h	9	3,2
	more than 4h	2	0,7
Failure to attend certain vaccination sessions	Afraid of injections	10	3,6
	Family constraints	79	28,2
	Long waiting wire	100	35,7
	Location too long	11	3,9
	Lack of money	7	2,5
	Lack of time	17	6,1
	Poor reception	32	11,4
	For lack of transport	12	4,3
	Family problems	12	4,3
Vaccination coverage	Fully vaccinated	74	26,4
	Incompletely vaccinated	194	69,3
	Never vaccinated	12	4,3

Most of the 192 mothers or babysitters (68.6%) spent 2 to 3 hours waiting for the vaccination service; 100 mothers (35.7%) missed some vaccination sessions due to queues, and were protective factors against non-vaccination or incomplete vaccination by a 95% CI for a risk α of 0.05.

9 Discussion:

9.1 Study limits:

The study was conducted in the seven urban health areas; the rest of the areas had also been excluded due to growing insecurity. This could be an important limitation to the generalizability of the present study's findings. There could also be a memory bias; mothers might not remember all the information. Nevertheless, the study revealed low vaccination coverage in two cities where geographical accessibility to health facilities is easy for most inhabitants. In other contexts, difficulties in accessing vaccination services were obstacles to vaccination. [1].

9.2 Vaccine completeness:

Our study found a vaccine completeness rate of 53.08% and a promptness rate of 46.92% in the Mopti health district in 2021, with 4.3% of children not vaccinated. Although this result is lower than the district data (69%), we note an improvement on the results of the EDS-V (45% in Bamako in 2018). [30]. However, the district coverage target of 95% has not been reached, with the exception of Pental, which is well above it. The risk of epidemics of targeted diseases is therefore high in the district. The vaccination card possession rate was 95.7%. This result is in line with most vaccination coverage surveys carried out in Bamako and Ségou in Mali [[10,11,24] and in Africa [[1,20]. Raising awareness and reinforcing the obligation to present a vaccination card before enrolling a child in kindergarten could improve the rate at which parents hold vaccination cards.

9.3 Vaccination coverage rate for children aged 0 to 23 months, by age group of mother:

Coverage varies according to the questioning of mothers or babysitters and the availability of vaccination cards. Mothers aged 25-35 had the highest number of incompletely vaccinated children (74), compared with (27) fully vaccinated children. This coverage represents a threat to children's herd immunity and the control of target diseases in the district. The factors associated with the incomplete vaccination of these children have been identified, and specific strategies need to be implemented to address them.

9.4 Immunization status of children by mother's level of education

Most of our children, including (82) incompletely vaccinated children and (36) fully vaccinated children, were born to mothers with primary education, compared with (7) never vaccinated children born to mothers with no schooling.

9.5   Factors associated with incomplete vaccination of children :

Waiting times of more than 1 hour at the vaccination center, missed vaccination sessions and shortages of vaccine consumables and doses were factors scientifically associated with incomplete vaccination of children aged 0 to 23 months. [20].

9.5.1   Waiting time at vaccination center greater than 1 hour :

This factor is linked to the organization of the vaccination post and session. It had already been identified in the 2012 vaccination coverage survey in Cameroon [20] as the main cause of children not being vaccinated.

9.5.2   Missed vaccination sessions:

This factor is due to long waiting times, poor reception, distance, not to mention lack of transport and family constraints.

9.5.3   Lack of consumables and vaccine doses:

This factor is also linked to poor estimation of needs or unmet needs from the Regional Health Department (DRS) to the Reference Health Center (CSREF) and the health area.

10 Conclusion:

Vaccination coverage in the Mopti health district in 2021 is below target. Health areas with children who have never been vaccinated have been identified.

Waiting times of more than 1 hour at the vaccination center, missed vaccination sessions and shortages of vaccine consumables and doses were factors leading to incomplete vaccinations for children aged 0 to 23 months.

11 Recommendations

Based on the results of our study, we make the following recommendations to help improve the health status of children aged 0 to 23 months:

Mopti Regional Health Department:

- o Avoid frequent antigen breaks
- o Place half-yearly orders for all Districts, taking buffer stock into account,
- o Fulfill District orders according to stock availability,
- o Provide Districts with good antigen storage capacity.

Mopti Health District:

- o Avoid frequent antigen breaks,
- o Place quarterly orders for all Aires de santé, taking buffer stock into account,
- o Fulfill orders from Aires de santé according to their vaccine target population.

District health areas :

- o Place monthly orders based on the monthly target population, taking buffer stock into account,
- o Use the media, religious leaders and husbands to sensitize mothers of children aged 0 to 23 months to continue attending vaccination services,
- o Enforce task allocation by health workers to improve communication with mothers of children aged 0 to 23 months,
- o Equal and equitable access to healthcare services in terms of vaccination.

Health area partners :

- o Strengthen the capacity of healthcare providers to educate mothers about vaccination,
- o Strengthen health care providers' capacity to reorganize health care and immunization.

12 References

1. Félicitée N, Hermann ND, Andreas C, Evelyn M, Guy W, Michel M, et al. Determinants and Reasons for Non-Complete Vaccination of Children Hospitalized in Two Pediatric Referral Hospitals in Yaoundé. 2018;19:8.

2 Faingezicht I, Avila-Aguerro ML, Cervantes Y, Fourneau M, Clemens SAC. Primary and booster vaccination with DTPw-HB/Hib pentavalent vaccine in Costa Rican children who had received a birth dose of hepatitis B vaccine. Rev Panam Salud Pública. Oct 2002;12:247-57.

3. Bos E, Batson A. Using Immunization Coverage Rates for Monitoring Health Sector Performance: Measurement and Interpretation Issues. Accessed 03/13/2022 at 11:16:53 [Internet]. Washington, DC: World Bank; 2000 Aug [cited 13 Mar 2022]. Available from: https://openknowledge.worldbank.org/handle/10986/13800

4. Id H. Factors associated with measles vaccination coverage in the Académie de Grenoble: comparison of areas with low and areas with high vaccination coverage in 2013. : 59.

5. Cohn A, Schuchat A. Vaccination coverage - an overview | ScienceDirect Topics [Internet]. [Cited March 27, 2022]. Available from: https://www-sciencedirect-com.translate.goog/topics/medicine-and-dentistry/vaccination-coverage?_x_tr_sl=en&_x_tr_tl=fr&_x_tr_hl=fr&_x_tr_pto=sc

6. K D. Issues of adequate penta 3 coverage in children aged 0-11 months in the Centre de Santé Communautaire et Universitaire de Konobougou, Mali. Mali Santé Publique. 20 Apr 2021;10(02):70-5.

7. Odusanya OO, Alufohai JE, Meurice FP, Clemens R, Ahonkhai VI. Short term evaluation of a rural immunization program in Nigeria. J Natl Med Assoc. Feb 2003;95(2):175-9.

8 Dimitri FY. Memoire Online - Etude des facteurs de réticence et de résistance à la vaccination anti-poliomyélite chez les populations de la commune de ZOGBODOMEY - Fabrice Dimitri Togla YEMADJE. Accessed 09/01/2022 at 12:42:57 [Internet]. Memoire Online. [Cited 9 Jan 2022]. Available at: https://www.memoireonline.com/06/09/2149/m_Etude-des-facteurs-de-reticence-et-de-resistance--la-vaccination-anti-poliomyelite-chez-les-populat0.html

9. Diop D, Sanicas M. Innovations in vaccinology: challenges and prospects for Africa. Pan Afr Med J. Apr 25, 2017;26:235.

10. Tounkara M. Evaluation de la couverture vaccinale chez les enfants âgés de 12 à 23 mois et les mères d'enfants âgés de 0 à 11 mois en commune I du district de Bamako en 2019 [Internet] [Thesis]. Université des Sciences, des Techniques et des Technologies de Bamako; 2020 [cited 13 nov 2021]. Available from: https://www.bibliosante.ml/handle/123456789/4021

11. Sangaré S, Sangho O, Doumbia L, Marker H, Sarro YDS, Dolo H, et al. Concordance of vaccination status and associated factors with incomplete vaccination: a household survey in the health district of Segou, Mali, 2019. Pan Afr Med J. 2021;40:102.

12   Saliou P. Vaccination and development in sub-Saharan Africa - Académie nationale de médecine | Une institution dans son temps [Internet]. [Cited March 13, 2022]. Available from: https://www.academie-medecine.fr/vaccination-et-developpement-en-afrique-sub-saharienne/

13.   Douba A, Aka LBN, Yao GHA, Zengbé-Acray P, Akani BC, Konan N. Sociodemographic factors associated with incomplete vaccination of children aged 12-59 months in six West African countries. Sante Publique (Bucur). Dec 31, 2015;27(5):723-32.

14   Decouttere C, De Boeck K, Vandaele N. Advancing sustainable development goals through immunization: to literature review. Glob Health. 26 August 2021;17:95.

15.   Duru CB, Iwu AC, Uwakwe KA, Diwe KC, Merenu IA, Emerole CA, et al. Assessment of Immunization Status, Coverage and Determinants among under 5-Year-Old Children in Owerri, Imo State, Nigeria. OALib. 2016;03(06):1-17.

16.   Maina LC, Karanja S, Kombich J. Immunization coverage and its determinants among children aged 12 - 23 months in a peri-urban area of Kenya. Pan Afr Med J. 2013;14:3.

17.   Islam T, Mandal S, Chouhan P. Influence of socio-demographic factors on coverage of full vaccination among children aged 12-23 months: a study in Indian context (2015-2016). Hum Vaccines Immunother. Dec 2, 2021;17(12):5226-34.

18.   Oku A, Oyo-Ita A, Glenton C, Fretheim A, Ames H, Muloliwa A, et al. Perceptions and experiences of childhood vaccination communication strategies among caregivers and health workers in Nigeria: A qualitative study. Ortiz JR, editor. PLOS ONE. Nov 8, 2017;12(11):e0186733.

19   Bourne PA, Kerr-Campbell MD. Determinants of self-rated private health insurance coverage in Jamaica. Health (N Y). 2010;02(06):541-50.

20.   Ba Pouth SFB, Kazambu D, Delissaint D, Kobela M. Vaccination coverage and factors associated with vaccine noncompleteness of children aged 12 to 23 months in the Djoungolo-Cameroon health district in 2012. Pan Afr Med J. Feb 4, 2014;17:91.

21   Kaboré A, Bachir GA, Ibrahim AS, Hervé H, Pauline Y. Prevalence and factors associated with missed vaccination opportunities (MVOs) in Niamey, Niger. 2021;5.

22.   Kirk K, McClair TL, Dakouo SP, Abuya T, Sripad P. Introduction of digital reporting platform to integrate community-level data into health information systems is feasible and acceptable among various community health stakeholders: A mixed-methods pilot study in Mopti, Mali. Accessed 13/03/2022 at 13:09:31. J Glob Health. 11:07003.

23.   Kaplan A, Botha ME, Dewey J, Shields P. Conceptual framework. In: Wikipedia [Internet]. 2020 [cited 22 Sep 2022]. Available from: https://fr.wikipedia.org/w/index.php?title=Cadre_conceptuel&oldid=178144527. Accessed 22/09/2022 at 18h28.

24.   Cissé YB. Study of factors influencing the quality of vaccination among children aged 0-11 months in the commune VI health district: case of the Yirimadio community health center. Accessed 03/27/2022 at 11:34:51 [Internet] [Thesis]. Université des Sciences, des

Techniques et des Technologies de Bamako; 2020 [cited March 27, 2022]. Available from: https://www.bibliosante.ml/handle/123456789/3796

25. Carine PMR. Professional master's degree in demography. : 166.

26 Gupta PK, Pore P, Patil U. Evaluation of Immunization Coverage in the Rural Area of Pune, Maharashtra, Using the 30 Cluster Sampling Technique. J Fam Med Prim Care. 2013;2(1):50-4.

27. Francis MR, Nuorti JP, Kompithra RZ, Larson H, Balraj V, Kang G, et al. Vaccination coverage and factors associated with routine childhood vaccination uptake in rural Vellore, southern India, 2017. Vaccine. May 21, 2019;37(23):3078-87.

28. UNICEF. Immunization schedule for children 0-11 months [Internet]. [Cited 22 Sep 2022]. Available from: https://www.unicef.org/drcongo/calendrier-vaccinal-enfants-rdc. Accessed 22/09/2022 at 18h50.

29. Giorgetta J. Vaccines in children: dates, reminders, the mandatory ones [Internet]. [Cited 22 Sep 2022]. Available at: https://sante.journaldesfemmes.fr/fiches-sante-du-quotidien/2540958-vaccins-enfant-dates-rappels-obligatoires-calendrier/Consulté on 22/09/2022 at 18h53.

30. INSTAT. Mali - Demographic and Health Survey 2018. Accessed 03.27.2022 at 20:54:39 [Internet]. [Cited March 27, 2022]. Available from: https://microdata.worldbank.org/index.php/catalog/3526

13.1 Mali enrolment consent form

Department of Public Health Teaching and Research

Research project title: Study of the factors influencing the low vaccination coverage of children aged 0 to 11 months and 12 to 23 months in the Mopti Health District in 2021 Principal investigator (Mali): Dr Seydou Amadou TRAORE

FMPOS protocol #: N°.../.../CE/FMPOS

Location: Mopti Health District and surrounding area, Mali, West Africa

Name and surname of participant: _______________________________________

Participant census ID number (if available): ______________________________

Information sheet

Aim of the study project

Study of the factors influencing the low vaccination coverage of children aged 0 to 11 months and 12 to 23 months in the Mopti Health District in 2021.

What you should know about this study

Immunization is recognized as one of the most effective measures for preventing mortality, morbidity and complications of infectious diseases in children. (3). Vaccination coverage indicates the proportion of the target population having received the required doses of a vaccine against a preventable disease (2). It is an important indicator of population health, and reflects the degree of susceptibility to vaccine-preventable diseases (3,4). It can also be used as a proxy to study the factors influencing accessibility to health services and vaccination-related interventions, providing a rapid study of the improvement or deterioration of health services. As high levels of immunization coverage are required to achieve the goals of reducing vaccine-preventable diseases, it is essential to monitor the various measures of immunization coverage on an ongoing basis.

We know that factors influencing vaccination coverage are rarely measured in the population as a whole, but rather in specific groups where vaccination is recommended. Where coverage is high, many children miss out on vaccination, leading to complications from infectious diseases. It is estimated that around 3 million deaths are prevented each year worldwide thanks to vaccination, and that, in addition, every year, it prevents almost 750,000 children from suffering serious physical, mental or neurological handicaps (7,8).

Why we ask you to participate

- ➢ You can take part in the study now if you are:
  - Mothers or babysitters of children aged 0 to 23 months, healthcare providers working in the field of vaccination.
  - Known resident of Mopti district or health area.
- ➢ You can't be in this study if you:
  - Have a condition that could affect your understanding of the study
  - Have a condition that could affect your safety and rights as a participant in this study or render you unable to properly participate in the study.

Study **procedures**

If you agree, you can take part in the study, and will then be included.

Risks and discomforts

Taking part in the study will take up some of your time, about 30 mm.

Alternative to study participation: Is not to participate in this study.

Benefits

You will not receive any direct benefit from your participation in the study, such as financial or material compensation. Your participation in the study is important and will help researchers understand how factors influence vaccination coverage in children aged 0 to 23 months.

Compensation: You will not receive any payment for lost study time.

Number of people in the study

Five health care providers and 140 mothers aged 0 to 23 months will be enrolled in the study.

Privacy

We will keep your health information confidential. All files containing information that could identify you will be kept in locked cabinets, but information such as your age and gender may be provided to researchers.

The people responsible for ensuring that the research is carried out correctly may look at your study file.

Future studies

Other investigators may wish to study our stored investigation files. In the event of future investigative needs, the files will be made available to them, without any information incriminating your private life.

Person to contact in case of need

If you require further information after the study, please contact the study team. They will ask the Principal Investigator : Dr Seydou Amadou TRAORE (Tel: +223 74093122).

You can also contact a member of the Ethics Committee of the Faculty of Medicine at

Pharmacie et Odontostomatologie (FMPOS) Prof Mahamadou DIAKITE, (Cell: 76 23 11 91) to answer any questions you may have about being part of this study and your rights as a research participant.

Consent form

I hereby acknowledge that I have read and understood the information provided in the information form concerning the above-mentioned study. I have had the opportunity to ask questions about this study and have received satisfactory answers. I understand the conditions of participation and the discomforts and benefits associated with my participation in this study. I understand that my participation is voluntary and that I may decide at any time to stop answering the survey questions without penalty.

I, the undersigned, voluntarily agree to participate in this study.

Participant's full name____

Participant's signature/fingerprint_______________________________________

Full name of person administering consent_______________________________

Signature of person administering consent________________________________

Date and place

13.2 Survey sheet :

Questionnaire for vaccinators

Name   of
respondent:...
Respondent
's position:...
Date   of   survey:..
Health   facility:... **I-**
Agents' knowledge of vaccination

 Q. 01 What are the EPI's target diseases?

Tuberculosis/__/   Diphtheria/__/   Pertussis/__/   Tetanus/__/   Poliomyelitis/__/
Measles/__/   Yellow   fever/__/   Hepatitis   B/__/   Hemophilus   b   infection/__/

Q. 02 At what age should children receive the following EPI vaccines?

BCG/VPO0 _______Birth Penta1, VPO1, PCV13 1, Rota1________6 weeks Penta2, VPO2,
PCV13 2, Rota2 _____10 weeks Penta3, VPO3, PCV13 3, Rota3, VPI1 ____14 weeks VAR1,
VAA MenAfrvac, VPI2_________9-11 months VAR2_________ 15-23 months

Q. 03 What are the contraindications for EPI vaccines?

....

....

Q. 04 Do   you   know   what   post   immunization   adverse   events   (P.I.A.E.)   are
?

Q. 05 Post-injection fever /__/ Post-injection local swelling /__/ Post-injection local redness
/__/ Post-injection local pain /__/ Injection-site abscess /__/ BCG-induced lymphadenitis /__/
Nothing /__/

Q. 06 Do you give any of the following information to the children's mothers or carers?

Possible side effects of vaccines Yes /__/ No /__/ Sometimes /_/

What to do in case of MAPI Yes /__/ no /__/ Sometimes /_/

Date of next appointment Yes /__/ No /__/ Sometimes /_/

Q. 07 If yes, what explanations do you give mothers about the need to continue
vaccination: ....

....

Q. 08 If yes, what information do you give to mothers about the possible side effects of vaccines: ....

....

Q. 09 In the event of MAPI, what would you do?

Reassure the mother /_/ Reassure and take charge of the child/_/ Do nothing/_/

Q. 10 How do you define missed opportunities?...

....

Q. 11 How do you define a case of abundance?...

....

Q. 12 How do you define a correctly and fully vaccinated child?.................

....

....

II - Program **management**

Q. 13 Have you received EPI training?

Formal training /__/ On-the-job training /__/

Q. 14 Have you received training in the following EPI areas?

Vaccine and injection material management Yes /__/ No /__/

Storage and handling of vaccines Yes /__/ No /__/

Logistics and cold chain maintenance Yes /__/ No /__/

Surveillance of EPI target diseases Yes /__/ No /__/

Injection safety and M.A.P.I. Yes /__/ No /__/

IEC and social mobilization in EPI Yes /__/ No /__/

EPI monitoring Yes /__/ No /__/

Vaccination techniques Yes /__/ No /__/

Q. 15 How many EPI supervisions did you receive in 2021? _________ supervision

Q. 16 Do you set vaccination coverage targets for this center? Yes /_/ No /_/

Q. 17 Can you calculate the vaccination coverage in this center?

If yes, do you have a graph for tracking purposes?   Yes /_/ No /_/

Q. 18 If No, why? Can't calculate /_/ Other /_/ No   answer /_/

Q. 19 Can you estimate the vaccine requirements for this center? Yes /_/ No /_/

Q. 20 If yes, what method do you use to calculate the center's vaccine requirements? By previous consumption /__/ By target population formula /__/ Other to specify /_/

Q. 21 How often do you stock up on vaccines?

Number: ....per week / month / quarter

Q. 22 Do you have EPI data collection media? Yes /_/ No /_/

Q. 23 If so, what media do you use?

Vaccination register /_/ Vaccine stock sheet /_/ Vaccine order booklet

/_/ vaccine movement book /_/

Q. 24 Will you be shutting down in 2021?   Yes /_/ No /_/

Q. 25 If yes, what are the causes of this cessation of activity?

No vaccine /_/ Break in the cold chain /_/ Period of strike by civil servants /_/

Others to be specified /_/

Q. 26 Do you organize social mobilization sessions in support of the EPI? Yes /_/ No /_/

Q. 27 If yes, how many sessions do you organize per month?........................

Q. 28 What steps have you taken to increase vaccination coverage?

Reduce drop-outs, missed opportunities and search for lost ones /_/

Raising mothers' awareness /_/ Doing nothing /_/

Q. 29 In your opinion, are vaccinators motivated? Yes /__/ No /__/

Q. 30 What do you suggest to encourage (motivate) vaccinators?

Reinforce staff /__/ Give a special bonus for vaccination /__/

Increase agents' salaries /__/ Congratulate agents /__/

Train agents /__/ Reinforce vaccination equipment /__/

No and signature of investigator :

Questionnaire for mothers of children aged 0 to 23 months

Health center:..   Survey date:...

I- Identification of mothers

Q. 31 Mother's age: 15 - 18 /__/ 19 - 24 /__/ 25 - 35 /__/ 35 - 49 /__/

Q. 32 Mother's level of education: None /_/ Primary /_/ Secondary /_/ Higher education /_/

Q. 33 Mother's occupation: Pupil /_/ Student /_/ Farmer /_/ Housewife /_/ Shopkeeper /_/

Craftswoman /_/ Other /_/

Q. 34 Marital status :

Single /_/ Living with a partner /_/ Widowed /_/ Divorced /_/ Married /_/

Q. 35 Child's full name: ....

Q. 36 Child's age in months: ....

Q. 37 Age in months /_/

Q. 38 Child immunization status:

Completely vaccinated /_/ Incompletely vaccinated /_/ Never vaccinated /_/

If possible, confirm vaccination status with vaccination record or injection sites.

Q. 39 If never vaccinated, what are the reasons? ....

....

....

II- Quality of vaccination services

Q. 40 Where do you go to vaccinate? Health center /_/ Elsewhere /_/

Q. 41 If you vaccinate elsewhere, what are the reasons?

....

Q. 42 What do you think of the welcome given by vaccinators?

Good /_/ acceptable /_/ Bad /_/

Q. 43 Justify your answer:

....

....

Q. 44 How much time do you spend at the vaccination center before you are

Vaccinated? < 1 h /_/ 1 - 2 h /_/ 2 - 3 h /_/ 3 - 4 h /_/ > 4 h /_/

Q. 45 How do you rate the waiting time at the vaccination service?

Normal/acceptable /_/ long /_/ other /_/

Q. 46 If other, please

specify:...

Q. 47 Do vaccinators tell you what diseases they are vaccinating your child against? Yes /_/ No /_/ Sometimes /_/

Q. 48 During vaccination sessions, do vaccinators talk to you about

Do you sometimes experience adverse reactions to this vaccine?

Yes /_/ No /_/ Sometimes /_/

Q. 49 Do vaccinators tell you when to come back for the rest of the vaccination?

Vaccination? Yes /_/ No /_/ Sometimes /_/ Other /_/

Q. 50 Are the center's vaccination days convenient for you?

Yes /_/ No /_/ Not always /_/ Other/_/ please specify:...

Q. 51 If other, please specify: ....

Q. 52 Are the vaccination hours at the center convenient for you?

Yes /_/ No /_/ Not always /_/ Other /_/ to be specified :...

Q. 53 If other, please specify:

....

Q. 54 Have you ever gone to the vaccination center and returned home?

Without being able to be vaccinated?

Yes /_/ No /_/ Sometimes /_/ Other /_/ please

specify:...

Q. 55 If other, please specify:...

....

Q. 56 If yes, what are the reasons?

No vaccines /_/ Vaccinator not present /_/ Poor reception /_/Other /_/

III- Mothers' vaccination knowledge

Q. 57 How are children vaccinated?

Against diseases /__/ Don't know /___/ Other to specify /___/

Q. 58 Do you think diseases can be prevented by traditional medicine?

Yes /_/ No /_/

Q. 59 Can vaccination be harmful to your child's health? Yes /__/ No /__/

Q. 60 If so, how?

....

....

Q. 61 In your opinion, what are the advantages of vaccination?

Vaccination protects children /_/ It's a good thing /_/ it's free /_/

We don't get sick anymore or do it less /_/ Other /_/ please specify ....

Q. 62 What limits vaccination for you?

Stinging /_/ its indirect costs /_/ rumors /_/ introducing in

the body a foreign substance /_/ its side effects /_/ the waiting time /_/ other /_/ please

specify:...

IV- Geographical accessibility for mothers of children aged 0 to 23 months

Q. 63 How do you rate the distance between your home and the center where you usually go

to vaccinate? Long /_/ Not long /_/Acceptable/_/Other /_/

Q. 64 If other, please

specify:...

Q. 65 Is distance a problem for you in getting to the center?

Vaccination?   Yes /_/ No /_/ Sometimes /_/ Other/_/

Q. 66 If other, please

specify:...

Q. 67 How much do you spend on average when you vaccinate a child?

Nothing /_/ < 200 FCFA /_/ 200-500FCFA /_/ 500- 1000 FCFA /_/ > 1000 CFA /_/

Q. 68 Is this bearable for you?   Yes /___/ No /___/

Q. 69 In your opinion, what are the reasons why you miss certain sessions?

Vaccination? Lack of time /_/ Household constraints /_/ Lack of means of transport /_/

Afraid of injections /_/ I'm not warned /_/ Poor reception /_/ Waiting line too long /_/ Agent

often not there /_/ Ignores need for vaccination /_/

Location too far /_/ Family problem /_/

Q. 70 How did you find out about vaccination?

Health center /___/ Administrative authorities /___/ Radio /___/ Print media /___/

Television /___/ Market/neighbours /___/ Husband /___/ Children /___/ Posters /___/

Banners /___/ Church/Mosque /___/ Traditional chiefs /___/ Red Cross volunteer /___/

Teachers/School /___/Don't know /___/

Q. 71 What do you suggest to vaccinate children regularly?

....

....

Q. 72 What would you suggest to encourage (motivate) vaccinators?

13.3 Gantt chart

Activities	Start date	End date	Nov 2021	Dec 2021	Jan. 2022	Feb. 2022	March 2022	Apr. 2022	May 2022	June 2022	July 2022	August 2022	Sept 2022
Literature reviews repository	25/11/ 2021	25/11/ 2021	■										
Methodology submission	25/12/ 2021	25/12/ 2021		■									
Deposit 1er Draft protocol	25/01/ 2022	25/01/ 2022			■								
Deposit 2nd Draft protocol	25/02/ 2022	25/02/ 2022				■							
Protocol validation	25/03/ 2022	25/03/ 2022					■						

Task	Start	End											
Field surveys	27/03/2022	31/05/2022		49		█	█	█					
Data analysis	01/06/2022	30/06/2022							█				
Memory correction	01/07/2022	15/08/2022								█			
Memory validation	16/08/2022	31/08/2022									█		
Dissertation defense	01/09/2022	30/09/2022										█	

13.4 Budget :

Designations	Unit	Number of days	Quantity	Price per unit	Total
Interviewer training					
Trainers	2	2	4	50000	200000
Investigators	3	5	15	20000	300000
Director	1	2	2	25000	50000
Maneuver	1	2	2	15000	30000
Total					580000
Consumables					
Notepad	3	1	3	1500	4500
Bic	3	1	3	100	300
Flap folders	3	1	3	1000	3000
Smartphones/Kobocollect	3	1	3	60000	180000
Paper reams	1	1	1	4000	4000
Connection kit	1	1	1	30000	30000
Total					221800
Room rental					
Tables and benches	8	2	16	40000	640000
Maintenance	1	2	2	10000	20000
Total					660000
Catering					
Coffee break	8	2	16	2500	40000
Lunch break	8	2	16	2500	40000
Drinking water	12	2	24	3250	78000
Water	24	2	48	8000	384000
Total					542000
Grand total					**2003800**

We close this budget at two million.

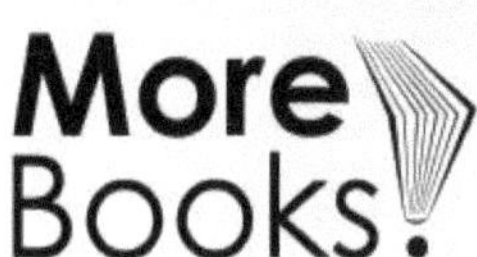

More
Books!

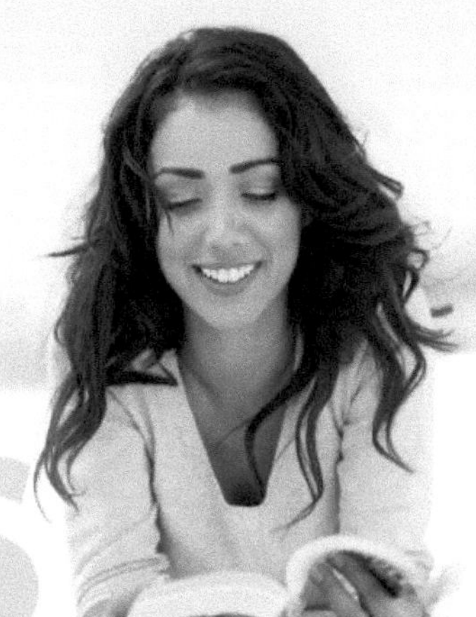

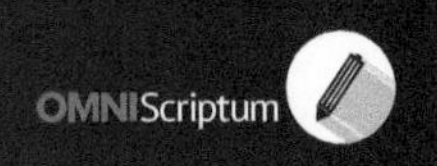

info@omniscriptum.com
www.omniscriptum.com
OMNIScriptum

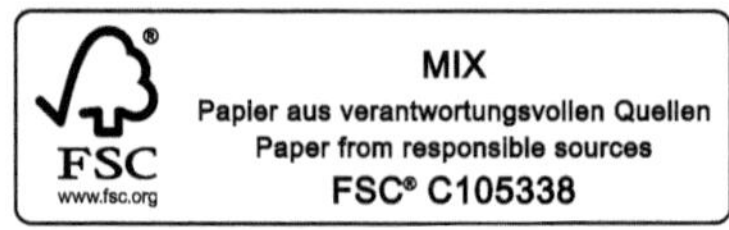

Printed by Books on Demand GmbH, Norderstedt / Germany